# From Couch Potato to Yoga Pro

## The Lazy Person's Step-by-Step Guide to Yoga, Improve Your Health, Fitness, and Well-being

Brawn Babe

# Table of Contents

# Introduction

Welcome to a journey that transforms couch-dwelling dreams into a tapestry of health, vitality, and unabashed laziness, a journey from being the ultimate couch potato to proudly donning the title of a Yoga Pro. If your idea of a workout involves searching for the remote, fear not! This isn't your typical yoga guide; it's a lazy person's ticket to a healthier, more flexible life without breaking a sweat.

Picture this: You, in the comfort of your favorite sagging couch cushions, discovering a world where yoga isn't just for the nimble, but for those who've perfected the art of Netflix marathons and snack binging. This isn't about contorting into pretzel-like shapes; it's about finding Zen while barely lifting a finger.

In the pages ahead, we'll debunk the myths that yoga is reserved for the hyper-motivated and spandex-clad. I'll let you in on a little secret, your journey to yoga greatness starts with a half-hearted stretch and a commitment to staying horizontal whenever possible.

But hey, don't just take my word for it. Imagine trading in that potato-chip-stained T-shirt for the effortless cool of a yoga guru, all while barely lifting your eyes from your favorite book or guilty-pleasure TV show. It's a transformation that's not just physical but one that'll stir your emotions, tickle your funny bone, and make you question why you didn't embark on this journey from the comfort of your couch sooner.

So, grab a cozy blanket, settle into your relaxation station, and let's embark on a quest that promises a healthier, happier you without losing sight of your commitment to the fine art of laziness. Welcome to "From Couch Potato to Yoga Pro", because who says enlightenment can't be achieved from the comfiest spot in the house? Let the adventure begin!

# Chapter 1

# Understanding Yoga for Lazy Beginners

## What is Yoga?

Welcome to the world of yoga, where the journey from being a couch potato to a yoga pro begins with understanding the essence of this ancient practice. In this chapter, we'll demystify the concept of yoga and explore how it can become a lazy person's perfect ally in the pursuit of better health, fitness, and overall well-being.

### *What is Yoga?*

Yoga is not just a series of complicated poses or a trendy fitness routine; it's a holistic approach to harmonizing the mind, body, and spirit. Imagine it as a magical recipe that blends physical postures, controlled breathing, meditation, and ethical principles to create a symphony of well-being.

### Practical Tips for Lazy Beginners:

**1. Start with the Basics:** Don't be intimidated by Instagram-worthy yoga poses. Begin with simple poses that allow your body to adjust gradually.

**2. Breathe Mindfully:** One of the fundamental aspects of yoga is conscious breathing. Take a few moments each day to focus on your breath, inhale positivity, exhale stress.

**3. Find Your Lazy Zone:** Yoga doesn't demand an hour of intense stretching. Identify your "lazy zone", those moments when you're lounging on the couch or sitting at your desk, and infuse them with simple yoga practices.

### *Actionable Advice:*

**1. Incorporate Yoga into Daily Activities:** Lazy yoga is all about integration. Practice subtle stretches while watching TV or perform seated yoga poses while working at your desk.

**2. Explore Online Resources:** There's a vast array of online platforms offering beginner-friendly yoga sessions. Find videos or apps that align with your lazy approach, allowing you to practice in the comfort of your home.

### *A Story to Connect:*

Meet Sarah, a self-proclaimed couch potato who discovered the power of lazy yoga. Initially skeptical, she started with basic stretches during her favorite TV shows. Gradually, Sarah found herself feeling more energized and less sluggish. Through this journey, she realized that yoga isn't reserved for the super-flexible;

it's for anyone willing to take small, lazy steps toward a healthier lifestyle.

**Breaking it Down:**
Yoga is like a buffet; you can choose what suits your taste. It's not about contorting into impossible poses; it's about finding peace in your own comfort zone. In the following chapters, we'll explore specific lazy poses and routines designed for beginners, making the journey from couch to yoga mat seamless.

In conclusion, understanding yoga is about embracing its simplicity and adapting it to your lazy lifestyle. So, let's take the first step on this journey together, unraveling the mysteries of yoga in a way that speaks to the lazy yogi in you.

# Benefits of Yoga for Lazy People

Congratulations on embarking on your lazy yoga journey! In this chapter, we'll delve into the delightful benefits that yoga can bring to those who prefer a more laid-back approach to fitness and well-being.

***The Lazy Person's Guide to Yoga Gains:***

**1. Increased Energy Levels:** Contrary to popular belief, yoga doesn't drain your energy; it replenishes it. Lazy yoga practices, even those as simple as deep breathing, can invigorate your body and mind, leaving you feeling more alive and alert.

**2. Improved Flexibility Without the Strain:** Forget the image of yogis contorting into pretzel-like shapes. Lazy yoga fosters gradual flexibility improvements, making daily movements easier and reducing the risk of injuries without pushing your body to extremes.

**3. Stress Reduction for the Lazily Stressed:** Life is hectic, but lazy yoga provides a sanctuary of calm. By incorporating mindfulness and relaxation techniques, you can melt away stress without breaking a sweat or leaving your comfort zone.

***Practical Tips for Lazy Yoga Benefits:***

**1. Start Small, Feel Big:** Lazy yoga is all about small, consistent efforts. Incorporate just a few minutes of yoga into your daily routine, and watch as the benefits accumulate over time.

**2. Mindful Resting:** Lazy people excel at resting, and yoga complements this skill. Learn the art of mindful resting through gentle poses and breathing exercises, promoting a sense of relaxation without the need for exhaustive workouts.

# Overcoming Common Myths and Misconceptions

**1. Myth:** Yoga is Only for the Flexible:
**Reality:** Lazy yoga welcomes all body types and fitness levels. It's not about touching your toes; it's about reaching for a healthier you, one lazy stretch at a time.

**2. Myth:** Yoga is Time-Consuming:
**Reality:** Lazy yoga is efficient. You don't need hours; a few minutes a day can make a significant impact. We'll explore time-friendly routines tailored for the perpetually lazy.

### 3. Myth: Yoga is Too Spiritual:
**Reality:** While yoga has spiritual roots, lazy yoga emphasizes the practical. You can enjoy the physical and mental benefits without delving into spiritual practices if it's not your cup of tea.

### A Lazy Success Story:
Meet Alex, a self-proclaimed "lazy achiever." Through lazy yoga, Alex found an unexpected surge in productivity and a newfound ability to tackle daily challenges with ease. The benefits of increased energy and reduced stress seamlessly fit into Alex's laid-back lifestyle.

# Chapter 2

# Creating Your Lazy Yoga Space

## Designing a Comfortable Yoga Space at Home

Welcome to the crucial step of establishing your lazy yoga haven. In this chapter, we'll explore the art of designing a comfortable yoga space at home, ensuring that your lazy yoga journey is not just effective but also enjoyable.

***Designing a Comfortable Yoga Space at Home:***

**1. Choosing the Right Location:**
- Identify a quiet and clutter-free area where you can escape the chaos of daily life.
- Consider natural light, if possible, to create a soothing atmosphere.

**2. Selecting Minimalistic Decor:**
- Opt for calming colors and simple decor to promote relaxation.

- Keep the space uncluttered, a minimalist approach enhances the sense of tranquility.

### 3. Investing in Comfortable Gear:
- Your lazy yoga space should be equipped with a comfortable mat, providing ample cushioning for your lazy stretches.
- Keep a cozy blanket or cushion nearby for added comfort during relaxation poses.

## *Practical Tips for Lazy Yoga Space Design:*

### 1. Adaptability is Key:
Your lazy yoga space doesn't need to be permanent. Choose an area that allows for easy setup and dismantling, accommodating your ever-changing lazy lifestyle.

### 2. Personal Touches Matter:
- Add elements that resonate with you, whether it's a favorite scented candle, soothing music, or a picture that brings you joy.
- Make it uniquely yours, creating a space you're drawn to.

## *Creating a Lazy Yoga Corner in Tight Spaces:*

### 1. Utilizing Corners and Nooks:

- If space is limited, carve out a corner or utilize an underused nook to establish your mini yoga sanctuary.
- Foldable yoga mats and compact accessories are perfect for optimizing small spaces.

**2. Incorporating Multi-Functional Furniture:**
- Choose furniture that serves dual purposes, such as a storage ottoman that doubles as a yoga prop storage.

*A Lazy Yoga Space Success Story:*

Meet Jamie, a busy professional with limited space. By transforming a corner of the living room into a lazy yoga oasis, Jamie seamlessly integrated short yoga sessions into the daily routine. The comfort and convenience of this personalized space made lazy yoga a consistent and enjoyable practice.

*Breaking it Down:*

Creating a comfortable yoga space at home is not just about aesthetics; it's about setting the stage for your lazy yoga success. As we move forward, you'll find that having a dedicated and inviting space makes it easier to transition from the couch to the yoga mat. So, let's dive into the practicalities of designing your ideal lazy yoga space and make it a sanctuary where your wellness journey can unfold effortlessly.

# Essential Yoga Gear for the Minimalist

Now that you've designed your lazy yoga space, it's time to explore the essential gear that will seamlessly integrate into your minimalist approach. In this chapter, we'll focus on the bare necessities, ensuring that your lazy yoga journey remains simple, practical, and, most importantly, devoid of unnecessary clutter.

### 1. The Lazy Yogi's Mat:
- Invest in a high-quality, non-slip yoga mat that provides adequate support for lazy stretches.
- Look for a mat that is easy to clean and can be stowed away effortlessly when not in use.

### 2. Multi-Functional Props:
- A versatile yoga block can be used to modify poses and enhance your lazy yoga experience.
- Consider a yoga strap for gentle stretching, especially if flexibility is a focus.

### 3. Comfortable Attire:
Choose loose, comfortable clothing that allows for easy movement. No need for elaborate yoga outfits, simplicity is key.

### 4. Ambient Lighting:

- If your lazy yoga space lacks natural light, opt for soft, ambient lighting to create a calming atmosphere.
- Minimalist lamps or candles can add a touch of tranquility without overwhelming the space.

## 5. Mindful Music or Soundscapes:
- Curate a playlist of calming tunes or nature sounds to enhance your lazy yoga sessions.
- Wireless earbuds can keep your experience personal without disturbing the minimalist ambiance.

### *Practical Tips for Minimalist Yoga Gear:*

## 1. Quality Over Quantity:
- Focus on a few high-quality items rather than accumulating numerous accessories.
- Prioritize gear that serves multiple purposes, eliminating the need for excess.

## 2. Storage Solutions:
- Explore minimalist storage options for your gear, such as wall-mounted hooks or foldable organizers.
- Keep your lazy yoga space clutter-free by stowing away gear when not in use.

### *A Minimalist Success Story:*
Meet Chris, a self-proclaimed minimalist. By carefully selecting a durable mat, a single yoga block, and a

versatile strap, Chris transformed a small corner into the perfect minimalist lazy yoga nook. The intentional choice of gear made the transition from couch to yoga mat seamless and clutter-free.

***Breaking it Down:***
Essential yoga gear for the minimalist is about quality, functionality, and purposeful choices. As you progress on your lazy yoga journey, remember that simplicity enhances the experience. In the following chapters, we'll delve into lazy poses and routines that require nothing more than the essentials, keeping your yoga practice refreshingly uncomplicated. So, let's embrace the minimalist spirit and dive into lazy yoga with the essentials that truly matter.

# Incorporating Lazy Yoga into Daily Routines

Congratulations on creating your cozy yoga space and gathering your essential gear. Now, let's explore the art of seamlessly integrating lazy yoga into your daily life.

### 1. Morning Lazy Yoga Rituals:
**Wake Up with Lazy Stretches:**
Start your day with a few gentle stretches in bed. Simple movements like reaching overhead or gentle twists can wake up your muscles and set a positive tone for the day.

**Mindful Morning Breathing:**
Before you even get out of bed, take a few moments for mindful breathing. Inhale deeply, fill your lungs, and exhale slowly. This helps oxygenate your body and clear your mind.

### 2. Lazy Yoga at the Desk:
**Seated Desk Yoga:**
Incorporate discreet yoga poses while sitting at your desk. Simple neck stretches, seated twists, and wrist rotations can relieve tension and boost your energy.

**Desk Yoga Breaks:**
Take short breaks throughout the day to stand up, stretch, and move. Even a minute of lazy yoga can refresh your mind and prevent stiffness.

### 3. *Evening Lazy Yoga Wind-Down:*
**TV Time Yoga:**
Make TV time productive by incorporating lazy yoga. Stretch your legs, practice seated poses, or even try balancing exercises during your favorite shows.

**Relaxing Bedtime Poses:**
Wind down before bed with a few relaxing poses. Gentle forward folds and calming stretches can signal to your body that it's time to relax.

## *Practical Tips for Lazy Yoga Integration:*

**1. Set Reminders:**
Use phone alarms or calendar reminders to prompt your lazy yoga sessions. Consistency is key, and gentle nudges can help establish a routine.

**2. Micro-Yoga Moments:**
Embrace micro-yoga throughout the day. Whether waiting for your coffee to brew or for a Zoom meeting to start, use these moments for quick stretches or mindful breaths.

### *A Lazy Integration Success Story:*
Meet Taylor, a busy professional with a hectic schedule. By incorporating lazy yoga into brief moments during the day, such as during phone calls or waiting for emails to load, Taylor transformed sedentary moments into opportunities for relaxation and rejuvenation.

# Chapter 3

# Gentle Poses for the Couch Potato Yogi

## Seated Yoga Poses for Beginners

Welcome to the heart of lazy yoga practice! In this chapter, we'll explore gentle seated yoga poses tailored for the couch potato yogi. These simple yet effective poses are designed to ease you into the world of yoga, providing a comfortable starting point for your journey to improved health and well-being.

**1. Easy Pose (Sukhasana):**
**How to:**
- Sit comfortably on the floor with your legs crossed.
- Rest your hands on your knees, palms facing up or down.
- Close your eyes and focus on your breath, allowing your spine to lengthen.

**Benefits:**
- Promotes groundedness and hip flexibility.
- Calms the mind and reduces stress.

### 2. Seated Forward Fold (Paschimottanasana):

**How to:**
- Sit with your legs extended in front of you.
- Hinge at your hips and reach towards your toes.
- Hold onto your shins, ankles, or feet, keeping your spine straight.

**Benefits:**
- Stretches the spine, hamstrings, and lower back.
- Relieves tension in the back and shoulders.

### 3. Cat-Cow Stretch (Marjarasana-Bitilasana):

**How to:**
- Come to a tabletop position with wrists under shoulders and knees under hips.
- Inhale, arch your back, and lift your head (Cow Pose).
- Exhale, round your spine, and tuck your chin to your chest (Cat Pose).

**Benefits:**
- Enhances spinal flexibility and mobility.
- Warms up the spine and releases tension.

### 4. Seated Side Stretch:

**How to:**
- Sit cross-legged or in Easy Pose.
- Inhale and raise your arms overhead.

- Exhale and gently lean to one side, stretching your torso.
- Inhale back to center, and repeat on the other side.

**Benefits:**
- Stretches the sides of the body and improves posture.
- Releases tension in the shoulders and neck.

### *Practical Tips for Seated Poses:*

### 1. Comfort is Key:
- Use a folded blanket or cushion under your sit bones if you find it hard to sit on the floor.
- Ensure your spine is comfortably aligned, avoiding unnecessary strain.

### 2. Mindful Breathing:
- Pay attention to your breath in each pose. Deep, rhythmic breathing enhances the benefits of the poses and promotes relaxation.

### *A Couch Potato Yogi's Success Story:*
Meet Alex, a self-professed couch potato who discovered the joy of seated yoga poses. By incorporating Easy Pose and Seated Forward Fold into TV time, Alex experienced a newfound sense of relaxation and increased flexibility.

***Breaking it Down:***
Seated yoga poses offer a gentle introduction to the world of lazy yoga. As you explore these beginner-friendly postures, remember that the journey is about comfort and progress, not perfection. In the following chapters, we'll build on these foundations and gradually introduce more poses, bringing you closer to your goal of becoming a yoga pro, one lazy stretch at a time.

# Reclining Poses for Relaxation

Now that we've explored seated poses, let's journey into the realm of relaxation with reclining yoga postures. These soothing poses are perfect for the couch potato yogi, offering deep relaxation and stress relief. Get ready to unwind and discover the lazy joy of reclining yoga.

## *1. Corpse Pose (Savasana):*

**How to:**
- Lie on your back with legs extended and arms by your sides, palms facing up.
- Close your eyes and focus on your breath.
- Allow your body to relax completely.

**Benefits:**
- Promotes deep relaxation and reduces stress.
- Enhances self-awareness and mindfulness.

## *2. Supine Bound Angle Pose (Supta Baddha Konasana):*

**How to:**
- Lie on your back and bring the soles of your feet together, allowing your knees to fall outward.
- Support your knees with cushions or props if needed.
- Relax your arms by your sides.

**Benefits:**
- Opens the hips and groin.
- Relieves tension in the lower back.

### *3. Legs Up the Wall Pose (Viparita Karani):*

**How to:**
- Sit close to a wall and swing your legs up, resting them against the wall.
- Keep your arms relaxed by your sides or on your abdomen.
- Close your eyes and breathe deeply.

**Benefits:**
- Alleviates tired legs and feet.
- Calms the nervous system and promotes relaxation.

### *4. Reclining Pigeon Pose:*

**How to:**
- Lie on your back with knees bent and feet flat on the floor.
- Cross your right ankle over your left knee, creating a figure-four shape.
- Thread your hands through and hold the back of your left thigh, gently pulling towards your chest.
- Repeat on the other side.

**Benefits:**
- Stretches the outer hips and glutes.

- Releases tension in the lower back.

## *Practical Tips for Reclining Poses:*

### 1. Create a Cozy Environment:
- Use a folded blanket or cushion under your head or knees for extra comfort.
- Play soft, calming music or use nature sounds to enhance the relaxation experience.

### 2. Extended Stay:
Allow yourself to stay in each reclining pose for at least 5-10 minutes, letting your body sink into deep relaxation.

### *A Relaxation Success Story:*
Meet Jamie, a busy parent who discovered the power of reclining yoga poses during moments of stress. By incorporating Savasana and Legs Up the Wall Pose into the bedtime routine, Jamie experienced a profound sense of calm and improved sleep quality.

### *Breaking it Down:*
Reclining yoga poses is your ticket to ultimate relaxation. As you explore these postures, focus on surrendering to the present moment and letting go of tension. In the upcoming chapters, we'll continue to build on these foundations, guiding you deeper into the lazy world of yoga relaxation. Get ready to melt into the serenity of reclining poses and embrace the tranquility they bring to your couch potato yogi journey.

# Incorporating Yoga into TV Time

Welcome to the delightful fusion of relaxation and entertainment, lazy yoga meets TV time. In this chapter, we'll explore how you can effortlessly integrate yoga into your favorite shows, transforming your TV time into a rejuvenating and mindful experience.

### 1. Seated Yoga Poses:

**Easy Pose with TV Twist:**
- Sit comfortably in Easy Pose while watching TV.
- Periodically twist gently to one side, then the other, engaging your core.

**TV Time Neck Stretches:**
- Sit comfortably and slowly tilt your head from side to side, bringing your ear towards your shoulder.
- Hold each stretch for a few breaths, releasing tension in your neck.

### 2. Reclining Yoga Poses:

**TV Time Legs Up the Wall:**
- Lie on your back with your legs resting up on the wall.
- Bring your attention to the TV while enjoying the benefits of this restorative pose.

**Reclining Pigeon Pose on the Couch:**
- Sit on the edge of your couch with one ankle crossed over the opposite knee.
- Gently hinge forward, feeling the stretch in your hips while keeping an eye on the screen.

### *3. TV Time Mindful Breathing:*

**Commercial Break Breath Awareness:**
- During commercial breaks, practice mindful breathing.
- Inhale deeply, exhale slowly and focus on your breath to center yourself.

### *Practical Tips for Incorporating Yoga into TV Time:*

**1. Choose Lazy-Friendly Shows:**
Opt for shows or movies that allow you to follow along with lazy yoga poses without missing crucial plot points.

**2. Create a TV Yoga Ritual:**
Designate specific shows or times for your TV yoga sessions, making it a ritual that enhances your viewing experience.

### *A TV Time Yoga Success Story:*
Meet Sarah, a dedicated TV enthusiast who turned her binge-watching sessions into opportunities for lazy yoga. By incorporating seated twists and reclining poses

during her favorite shows, Sarah found a perfect balance between relaxation and entertainment.

**Breaking it Down:**
Incorporating yoga into TV time is a win-win – you get to enjoy your favorite shows while reaping the benefits of gentle yoga. As we move forward, you'll discover more ways to seamlessly integrate lazy yoga into various aspects of your daily life. So, grab your remote and get ready to explore the lazy yoga possibilities that await during your next TV session.

# Chapter 4

# Lazy Yoga Sequences for Busy Schedules

## Quick and Effective Yoga Routines

Welcome to the chapter designed for the busiest of couch potatoes, those who crave the benefits of yoga but have minutes, not hours. In this chapter, we'll explore short and effective lazy yoga sequences tailored for the time-strapped, ensuring that you can infuse the magic of yoga into even the most hectic schedules.

### *1. Energizing Morning Flow:*

**Mountain Pose to Forward Fold:**
- Stand with feet hip-width apart, inhale arms overhead.
- Exhale and hinge at the hips, reaching towards the floor.
- Repeat for 5 cycles, awakening your body.

**Downward Dog to Upward Dog:**
- From a plank position, push back into Downward Dog.
- Inhale, shift to Upward Dog, opening your chest.

- Repeat 5 times to build strength and flexibility.

## *2. Desk Yoga for Midday Refresh:*

### Seated Cat-Cow Stretch:
- Sit comfortably in your chair.
- Inhale, arch your back, and lift your chest.
- Exhale, around your spine.
- Repeat for 3-5 cycles to release tension.

### Chair Pigeon Pose:
- While seated, cross your right ankle over your left knee.
- Sit tall and lean forward slightly, feeling a stretch in your hip.
- Hold for 30 seconds, then switch sides.

## *3. Relaxing Evening Routine:*

### Child's Pose to Thread the Needle:
- Begin in Child's Pose, reaching your arms forward.
- Slide your right arm under your left, resting on your shoulder.
- Hold for 30 seconds, then switch sides.

### Legs Up the Wall:
- Lie on your back and extend your legs up the wall.
- Relax for 2-5 minutes, focusing on deep breaths.

***Practical Tips for Quick Yoga Routines:***

## 1. Consistency Over Duration:
- Aim for short, daily sessions rather than occasional lengthy ones.
- Even 10 minutes of lazy yoga can make a significant impact.

## 2. Mindful Breathing:
Integrate conscious breathing into each sequence, enhancing the calming benefits of your lazy yoga practice.

*### A Busy Yogi Success Story:*
Meet Alex, a professional juggling work and family commitments. By incorporating quick yoga routines during breaks, Alex experienced improved focus, reduced stress, and a newfound sense of balance.

*### Breaking it Down:*
Quick and effective yoga routines are your secret weapon for weaving lazy yoga into the busiest of days. As we move forward, you'll discover more bite-sized sequences tailored to your schedule, ensuring that even the most time-strapped couch potatoes can enjoy the benefits of a consistent lazy yoga practice. Get ready to squeeze in moments of relaxation and rejuvenation, one short routine at a time.

# Desk Yoga for the Office Couch Potato

Welcome to the chapter designed specifically for those navigating the demands of the office while maintaining their couch potato status. In this chapter, we'll explore Desk Yoga, a series of gentle and discreet yoga poses that can be seamlessly integrated into your workday, helping you stay relaxed and rejuvenated even amid office chaos.

## 1. Seated Desk Stretches:

**Neck Rolls:**
- Sit tall and drop your chin to your chest.
- Slowly roll your head to one side and then to the other.
- Repeat for 30 seconds, releasing tension in the neck.

**Shoulder Shrugs:**
- Inhale, lifting your shoulders towards your ears.
- Exhale, rolling them back and down.
- Repeat for 1 minute to alleviate shoulder tension.

## 2. Chair Yoga Poses:

**Seated Forward Fold:**
- Sit on the edge of your chair with your feet flat on the floor.

- Hinge at your hips, reaching towards your toes.
- Hold for 30 seconds, stretching your spine.

**Chair Pigeon Pose:**
- Sit tall and cross your right ankle over your left knee.
- Gently press on your right knee to deepen the stretch.
- Hold for 30 seconds, then switch sides.

### *3. Mindful Breathing at Your Desk:*

**Box Breathing:**
- Inhale for a count of 4.
- Hold your breath for a count of 4.
- Exhale for a count of 4.
- Repeat for 2 minutes to calm the nervous system.

### *Practical Tips for Desk Yoga:*

**1. Incorporate Regular Breaks:**
- Set reminders to take short breaks throughout the day.
- Use these breaks for quick desk yoga sessions.

**2. Modify for Privacy:**
- Choose poses that can be discreetly done in your office space.
- Close your office door or find a quiet corner for a few moments of yoga privacy.

### An Office Yogi Success Story:
Meet Taylor, a corporate professional with a demanding schedule. By integrating Desk Yoga into short breaks, Taylor experienced reduced stress levels and increased focus during work hours.

### Breaking it Down:
Desk Yoga is your secret weapon for maintaining your lazy yoga routine amid a bustling workday. As we move forward, you'll discover more ways to seamlessly blend lazy yoga into different aspects of your daily life. Get ready to transform your workspace into a haven of relaxation and well-being, one discreet pose at a time.

# Yoga Nidra for Ultimate Relaxation

Enter the realm of ultimate relaxation with Yoga Nidra, a powerful practice that allows the couch potato yogi to experience deep relaxation and rejuvenation. In this chapter, we'll explore the art of Yoga Nidra, guiding you through a journey of profound restfulness even in the busiest of schedules.

### *Understanding Yoga Nidra:*

Yoga Nidra, often referred to as yogic sleep, is a state of conscious relaxation that guides you to the edge of sleep while keeping the mind alert. It's a practice that promotes deep restorative rest, making it an ideal addition to the lazy yogi's toolkit.

### *1. Finding a Comfortable Position:*

**Lie Down Comfortably:**
- Find a quiet and comfortable space to lie down on your back.
- Use a blanket or eye mask if needed, ensuring you're warm and at ease.

### *2. Guided Relaxation:*

**Body Scan:**
- Close your eyes and bring your attention to each part of your body, starting from your toes and moving up to the crown of your head.

- Release tension with each breath, letting go of any tightness or discomfort.

**Breath Awareness:**
- Focus on your breath, allowing it to flow naturally.
- Follow the sensation of inhaling and exhaling, bringing your attention back if the mind starts to wander.

### *3. Visualization:*

**Create a Relaxing Scene:**
- Imagine a tranquil place, such as a beach or a forest.
- Engage your senses, envisioning the sights, sounds, and sensations of this peaceful environment.

### *4. Intention Setting:*

**Set a Positive Intention:**
- Reflect on a positive affirmation or intention for your well-being.
- Repeat this affirmation silently, reinforcing a positive mindset.

### *Practical Tips for Yoga Nidra:*

### 1. Time Considerations:

- A session of Yoga Nidra can range from 10 minutes to an hour.
- Tailor the duration based on the time available and your personal preferences.

**2. Consistency is Key:**
- Practice Yoga Nidra regularly, preferably at the same time each day or night.
- Consistency enhances its effectiveness over time.

***A Yoga Nidra Success Story:***
Meet Alex, a couch potato yogi facing high stress levels. By incorporating Yoga Nidra into the nightly routine, Alex experienced improved sleep quality, reduced anxiety, and an overall sense of well-being.

***Breaking it Down:***
Yoga Nidra is your gateway to ultimate relaxation, allowing you to tap into the profound benefits of restfulness and mindfulness. As we move forward, you'll discover more lazy yoga practices that enhance your well-being, bringing you closer to the goal of a harmonious and balanced lifestyle. Get ready to embark on a journey of deep relaxation with Yoga Nidra, the lazy yogi's path to ultimate tranquility.

*A powerful practice that allows the couch potato yogi to experience deep relaxation and rejuvenation.*

# Chapter 5

# Overcoming Laziness and Building Consistency

## Motivational Tips for Lazy Yogis

Congratulations on your lazy yoga journey so far! In this chapter, we'll address a common hurdle faced by couch potato yogis, overcoming laziness and building the consistency needed for a sustainable practice. Let's dive into motivational tips to keep your lazy yoga routine on track.

### 1. Set Realistic Goals:

**Start Small, Dream Big:**
- Begin with achievable goals that fit your current lifestyle.
- Gradually increase the intensity and duration as your lazy yoga journey progresses.

### 2. Find Joy in the Practice:

**Discover What You Love:**
- Identify lazy yoga poses and routines that bring you joy.

- When you enjoy your practice, laziness transforms into enthusiasm.

### 3. Create a Routine:

**Establish a Lazy Yoga Schedule:**
- Set aside dedicated time for lazy yoga each day.
- Whether it's in the morning, during breaks, or before bedtime, consistency is key.

### 4. Accountability Partners:

**Lazy Yoga Buddies:**
- Share your lazy yoga goals with a friend or family member.
- Having a buddy can provide motivation and accountability.

### 5. Track Your Progress:

**Celebrate Small Wins:**
- Keep a lazy yoga journal to track your progress.
- Celebrate each small achievement to stay motivated.

### 6. Mix it Up:

**Lazy Variety:**
- Keep your lazy yoga routine interesting by trying different poses and sequences.

- Variety prevents boredom and sparks renewed interest.

## 7. Remind Yourself of the Benefits:

**Reflect on the Positives:**
- Regularly remind yourself of the benefits you've experienced.
- Whether it's increased energy, reduced stress, or improved flexibility, focus on the positive outcomes.

## 8. Embrace Imperfection:

**Lazy Days Happen:**
- Accept that there will be days when you feel extra lazy.
- Embrace imperfection, and don't let occasional setbacks discourage you.

## 9. Create a Relaxing Environment:

**Yoga Nook Bliss:**
- Designate a calming space for your lazy yoga practice.
- A tranquil environment encourages consistency and helps overcome the inertia of laziness.

## 10. Be Kind to Yourself:

**Lazy Self-Compassion:**

- Approach your lazy yoga journey with kindness.
- Be patient with yourself, and understand that progress takes time.

### A Motivational Success Story:

Meet Jamie, a once-reluctant lazy yogi who struggled with consistency. By implementing these motivational tips, Jamie transformed from occasional practices to a daily routine, experiencing increased energy and a sense of accomplishment.

### Breaking it Down:

Building consistency in lazy yoga is about finding inspiration and joy in your practice. As we move forward, you'll discover more motivational tips and lazy yoga strategies to keep you on the path of well-being. Get ready to overcome laziness, embrace consistency, and continue your journey toward becoming a true yoga pro, the lazy way.

# Setting Realistic Goals

Welcome to the pivotal chapter where we'll dive into the essential steps of setting realistic goals and establishing a consistent lazy yoga routine. This foundation will propel you forward on your journey to becoming a seasoned couch potato yogi.

### *1. Assess Your Current Lifestyle:*

**Honest Self-Reflection:**
- Evaluate your daily schedule, considering work, family commitments, and leisure time.
- Understand your energy levels at different times of the day.

### *2. Start Small, Dream Big:*

**Micro-Goals for Macro Success:**
- Begin with easily attainable goals, such as a five-minute lazy yoga session.
- Gradually increase the duration and intensity as you build consistency.

### *3. Define Your Lazy Yoga Objectives:*

**Personalize Your Journey:**
- Clarify why you're embarking on this lazy yoga adventure. Is it for relaxation, flexibility, or overall well-being?

- Tailor your goals to align with your unique intentions.

### 4. Set Realistic Time Commitments:

**Quality Over Quantity:**
- Understand that a brief, focused lazy yoga routine can be more beneficial than a lengthy, sporadic one.
- Aim for a duration that suits your schedule, even if it's just a few minutes each day.

### 5. Establish a Lazy Yoga Schedule:

**Consistency is Key:**
- Designate specific times for your lazy yoga practice each day.
- Whether it's in the morning, during lunch breaks, or before bedtime, having a set routine fosters consistency.

### 6. Gradual Progression:

**Level Up at Your Pace:**
- As you become comfortable with your routine, gradually add new poses or extend the duration.
- Allow your lazy yoga journey to evolve naturally.

### 7. Mix and Match:

**Variety Keeps it Fresh:**

- Experiment with different lazy yoga poses and sequences.
- A diverse routine prevents monotony and keeps you engaged.

## 8. Embrace Flexibility:

### Adapt to Life's Changes:
- Understand that your routine may need adjustments during busy periods.
- Embrace flexibility without abandoning your lazy yoga commitment.

## 9. Track Your Progress:

### Celebrate Milestones:
- Keep a lazy yoga journal to document your achievements.
- Celebrate both small and significant milestones to stay motivated.

## 10. Seek Support:

### Lazy Yoga Community:
- Connect with other lazy yogis, either online or in your local community.
- Share experiences, tips, and encouragement to enhance motivation.

***A Goal-Setting Success Story:***
Meet Alex, a busy professional who initially struggled with consistency. By setting small, achievable goals and establishing a realistic routine, Alex transformed into a dedicated couch potato yogi, experiencing increased energy and a sense of accomplishment.

***Breaking it Down:***
Setting realistic goals and establishing a lazy yoga routine is the bedrock of a successful journey. As we move forward, you'll discover more tools and strategies to navigate the challenges of laziness and build a consistent practice that aligns seamlessly with your lifestyle. Get ready to embrace the power of achievable goals and establish a lazy yoga routine that becomes an integral part of your daily life.

# Chapter 6

# Yoga for Health and Well-being

## Improving Flexibility and Mobility

Welcome to a chapter dedicated to enhancing your health and overall well-being through the transformative power of lazy yoga. In this segment, we'll explore the specific benefits of improving flexibility and mobility, uncovering how these elements contribute to your journey of becoming a healthier and more vibrant couch potato yogi.

### *1. The Significance of Flexibility:*

**A Gateway to Well-being:**
- Flexibility is more than just touching your toes; it's about functional freedom in your movements.
- Improved flexibility can alleviate stiffness, enhance posture, and contribute to an overall sense of ease.

### *2. Lazy Yoga Poses for Flexibility:*

**Downward Dog Stretch:**
- Begin in a tabletop position and lift your hips towards the ceiling, forming an inverted V-shape.
- Pedal your feet to stretch the calves and hamstrings gradually.

**Forward Fold (Uttanasana):**
- Stand with feet hip-width apart and hinge at your hips, reaching towards the floor.
- Allow gravity to gently pull you deeper into the stretch.

### 3. The Role of Mobility in Health:

**Freedom of Movement:**
- Mobility refers to the range of motion your joints can achieve actively.
- Improved mobility supports daily activities, prevents injury, and enhances your overall quality of life.

### 4. Lazy Yoga Poses for Mobility:

**Seated Hip Opener:**
- Sit with your legs crossed and gently press your knees towards the floor.
- This pose enhances hip mobility, particularly beneficial for those with sedentary lifestyles.

**Twisting Chair Pose:**

- From a standing position, sit back into a chair pose.
- Twist your torso to one side, then the other, promoting mobility in the spine and hips.

## 5. The Lazy Yogi's Approach to Progress:

### Consistency Over Intensity:
- Regular, gentle practice trumps sporadic intense sessions.
- Lazy yoga focuses on gradual improvement, preventing strain or injury.

## 6. Mindful Stretching for Well-being:

### Conscious Awareness in Movement:
- Pair your lazy yoga poses with mindful breathing to deepen the sense of relaxation and release.
- Each stretch becomes an opportunity to cultivate a mind-body connection.

## 7. Incorporating Flexibility and Mobility into Lazy Routines:

### Seamless Integration:
- As you progress on your lazy yoga journey, infuse flexibility and mobility exercises into your daily routines.
- Stretch during TV time, incorporate movements during breaks, and find moments to indulge in mindful stretches.

### 8. Celebrating Small Victories:

**Acknowledge Progress:**
- Celebrate the incremental improvements in your flexibility and mobility.
- Recognize that each lazy yoga session contributes to your overall health and well-being.

### A Flexibility and Mobility Success Story:
Meet Taylor, who initially faced stiffness from prolonged office hours. By incorporating lazy yoga poses designed for flexibility and mobility, Taylor experienced increased comfort, reduced stiffness, and a newfound sense of physical freedom.

### Breaking it Down:
Improving flexibility and mobility through lazy yoga is a holistic approach to enhancing your health and well-being. As we move forward, you'll delve deeper into poses and routines specifically crafted to address various aspects of your physical and mental health. Get ready to unfold the full potential of lazy yoga, embracing a more flexible, mobile, and vibrant version of yourself.

# Yoga for Stress Reduction

In this chapter, we'll explore the profound benefits of lazy yoga in alleviating stress and promoting mental well-being. As a couch potato yogi, you'll discover how simple yet effective practices can help you unwind, release tension, and cultivate a calmer state of mind.

## *1. Understanding the Stress-Relief Power of Yoga:*

### Mind-Body Harmony:
- Lazy yoga provides a holistic approach to stress reduction by combining gentle movement, mindful breathing, and relaxation techniques.
- The calming effects of yoga extend beyond the physical body, promoting mental and emotional well-being.

## *2. Lazy Yoga Poses for Stress Reduction:*

### Child's Pose (Balasana):
- Kneel on the mat, sit back on your heels, and extend your arms forward.
- This restful pose helps release tension in the back and shoulders, inducing a sense of calm.

### Corpse Pose (Savasana):
- Lie on your back with legs extended and arms by your sides, palms facing up.

- Savasana allows for deep relaxation, calming the nervous system and reducing stress levels.

## 3. Mindful Breathing Techniques:

### Diaphragmatic Breathing:
- Place one hand on your chest and the other on your abdomen.
- Inhale deeply through your nose, allowing your abdomen to rise, then exhale slowly.
- Diaphragmatic breathing activates the relaxation response, easing stress and anxiety.

### Alternate Nostril Breathing (Nadi Shodhana):
- Sit comfortably, close your right nostril with your thumb, and inhale through the left nostril.
- Close the left nostril with your ring finger and exhale through the right nostril.
- This technique balances the nervous system, promoting a sense of calm.

## 4. Incorporating Stress Relief into Daily Routines:

### Morning Mindful Breathing Ritual:
- Start your day with a few minutes of mindful breathing.
- Inhale positivity, exhale stress, setting a positive tone for the day.

### Desk Yoga Stress Breaks:

- Take short breaks during work to practice stress-relief poses.
- Incorporate gentle stretches and breathing exercises to refresh your mind.

## 5. *The Lazy Yogi's Approach to Stress Management:*

### Consistent Practice for Lasting Effects:
- Regular, lazy yoga practice builds resilience to stress over time.
- Even short sessions contribute to a cumulative effect, creating a buffer against daily stressors.

## 6. *Mindfulness in Motion:*

### Present Moment Awareness:
- Engage in lazy yoga with full attention to the present moment.
- Allow gentle movements and breath awareness to anchor you in the here and now, reducing stress associated with future concerns.

## 7. *Celebrating Inner Peace:*

### Acknowledge Your Progress:
- Celebrate the moments of tranquility and peace that arise during and after your lazy yoga sessions.
- Recognize the value of these moments in your overall stress reduction journey.

***A Stress-Relief Success Story:***
Meet Jamie, a couch potato yogi who battled daily stress from a demanding job. Through consistent lazy yoga practice, incorporating stress-relief poses and mindful breathing, Jamie experienced a significant reduction in stress levels, leading to improved overall well-being.

***Breaking it Down:***
Lazy yoga offers a sanctuary of peace amid a hectic world. As we continue on this journey, you'll uncover more stress-reducing techniques and discover how the gentle art of lazy yoga can be a powerful tool in cultivating a calmer, more resilient mind. Get ready to embrace the tranquility and balance that lazy yoga brings to your life.

# Lazy Yoga for Better Sleep

Welcome to a chapter dedicated to the essential role lazy yoga plays in promoting restful and rejuvenating sleep. As a couch potato yogi, you'll explore how gentle yoga practices can create a calming bedtime routine, helping you unwind, release tension, and prepare your body and mind for a night of quality sleep.

## *1. The Connection Between Lazy Yoga and Better Sleep:*

**Calming the Nervous System:**
- Lazy yoga encourages relaxation, calming the nervous system and signaling to the body that it's time to wind down.
- This transition from daily activities to a state of rest is crucial for improved sleep quality.

## *2. Lazy Yoga Poses for Bedtime Bliss:*

**Legs Up the Wall Pose (Viparita Karani):**
- Lie on your back and extend your legs up the wall.
- This pose promotes relaxation, relieves tired legs, and facilitates the gentle flow of energy.

**Reclining Butterfly Pose (Supta Baddha Konasana):**
- Lie on your back and bring the soles of your feet together, allowing your knees to fall outward.

- A restful pose that opens the hips and encourages a sense of surrender.

### 3. Gentle Stretching to Release Tension:

**Seated Forward Bend (Paschimottanasana):**
- Sit with legs extended, hinge at the hips, and reach towards your toes.
- This forward bend stretches the spine, and hamstrings, and helps release tension.

**Child's Pose (Balasana):**
- Kneel on the mat, sit back on your heels, and extend your arms forward.
- Child's Pose gently stretches the back and promotes a sense of tranquility.

### 4. Breath Awareness for a Restful Mind:

**Counted Breath Relaxation:**
- Lie comfortably on your back and focus on your breath.
- Inhale for a count of four, exhale for a count of six.
- This breath pattern slows down the nervous system, inducing relaxation.

### 5. Creating a Bedtime Lazy Yoga Routine:

**Consistent Wind-Down Rituals:**
- Establish a lazy yoga routine before bedtime.

- Consistency signals to your body that it's time to transition into sleep mode.

**Screen-Free Zone:**
- Create a screen-free zone at least 30 minutes before bedtime.
- Use this time for lazy yoga, allowing your mind to unwind from the day's activities.

## 6. Mindful Relaxation for Sound Sleep:

**Body Scan Meditation:**
- Lying in bed, brings attention to each part of your body, releasing tension.
- Allow your awareness to move from head to toe, promoting a state of deep relaxation.

## 7. The Lazy Yogi's Approach to Sleep Enhancement:

**Quality Over Quantity:**
- Aim for a short and focused lazy yoga routine before bed.
- Quality practice is key to reaping the sleep-enhancing benefits.

## 8. Celebrating Sweet Dreams:

**Acknowledge Improved Sleep:**
- Celebrate nights of deep, restful sleep as a result of your bedtime lazy yoga routine.

- Recognize the positive impact on your overall health and well-being.

### A Better Sleep Success Story:
Meet Alex, a couch potato yogi who struggled with insomnia. Through the consistent practice of bedtime lazy yoga, incorporating gentle poses and relaxation techniques, Alex experienced a significant improvement in sleep quality, leading to increased daytime energy and focus.

### Breaking it Down:
Lazy yoga becomes a soothing lullaby for your body and mind, paving the way for better sleep. As we journey forward, you'll uncover more bedtime rituals and lazy yoga practices designed to enhance the quality of your rest. Get ready to embrace the serenity of a bedtime lazy yoga routine, inviting sweet dreams and a rejuvenated morning ahead.

# Chapter 7

# Nutritional Support for the Lazy Yogi

## Simple and Healthy Eating Habits

In this chapter, we'll explore the symbiotic relationship between lazy yoga and nutrition. As a couch potato yogi, you'll discover how adopting simple and healthy eating habits can complement your lazy yoga practice, providing the necessary fuel for energy, recovery, and overall well-being.

### *1. The Lazy Yogi's Balanced Plate:*

**Embracing Nutrient Diversity:**
- Strive for a well-balanced plate that includes a variety of colors, textures, and nutrient-dense foods.
- Incorporate a mix of whole grains, lean proteins, healthy fats, and an abundance of fruits and vegetables.

### *2. Mindful Eating for Digestive Harmony:*

**Savoring Each Bite:**

- Practice mindful eating, savoring the flavors and textures of your food.
- Eating with awareness promotes better digestion and allows you to tune in to your body's hunger and fullness cues.

### 3. Pre- and Post-Lazy Yoga Nutrition:

**Pre-Lazy Yoga Fuel:**
- Consume a light and balanced meal or snack before your lazy yoga session.
- Opt for easily digestible foods such as fruits, yogurt, or whole-grain toast.

**Post-Lazy Yoga Recovery:**
- Replenish your body with a combination of protein and carbohydrates after your lazy yoga practice.
- This aids in muscle recovery and replenishes energy stores.

### 4. Hydration as a Foundation:

**Water, the Elixir of Life:**
- Stay well-hydrated throughout the day.
- Water supports overall bodily functions, aids digestion, and enhances the benefits of your lazy yoga practice.

### 5. Simplicity in Snacking:

**Nutritious Snack Options:**
- Choose easy and wholesome snacks for sustained energy.
- Examples include nuts, seeds, fresh fruit, or yogurt.

### *6. Lazy Meal Planning:*

**Effortless Healthy Options:**
- Plan simple and nutritious meals that require minimal preparation.
- Batch-cooking and one-pot meals can be lifesavers for the busy couch potato yogi.

### *7. Superfoods for Lazy Yogis:*

**Incorporating Nutrient Powerhouses:**
- Include superfoods like berries, leafy greens, and nuts in your diet.
- These nutrient-dense foods contribute to overall health and vitality.

### *8. Mind-Body Connection in Eating:*

**Listen to Your Body:**
- Pay attention to how different foods make you feel.
- Your body's response can guide you in making food choices that support your well-being.

### *9. Lazy Yogi's Hygge Dining:*

**Creating a Cozy Eating Environment:**
- Establish a relaxed and comfortable space for meals.
- Enjoying your food in a tranquil environment enhances the dining experience.

### *10. Celebrating Nutritional Harmony:*
**Acknowledge Nourishment Achievements:**
- Celebrate the small victories in adopting healthy eating habits.
- Recognize the positive impact on your energy levels, mood, and overall lazy yoga experience.

### *A Nutritional Harmony Success Story:*
Meet Taylor, a couch potato yogi who transformed eating habits to align with a lazy yoga lifestyle. By embracing simple, nutritious choices, Taylor experienced increased energy levels, improved focus, and enhanced well-being.

### *Breaking it Down:*
Nutritional support is the silent partner in your lazy yoga journey, enhancing the benefits of your practice and contributing to your overall health. As we move forward, you'll delve deeper into the symbiosis between lazy yoga and nutrition, uncovering more ways to fuel your body and mind for a harmonious and balanced lifestyle. Get ready to celebrate the delicious and nutritious journey of the lazy yogi's plate.

# Lazy Yogi Snack Ideas

Snacking as a lazy yogi doesn't have to be complicated or time-consuming. In this section, we'll explore simple, nutritious, and delicious snack ideas that perfectly complement your laid-back approach to yoga and wellness.

### 1. Nut and Seed Mix:
- Create a custom mix of almonds, walnuts, pumpkin seeds, and sunflower seeds.
- Packed with protein, healthy fats, and a variety of nutrients to keep you energized.

### 2. Greek Yogurt Parfait:
- Layer Greek yogurt with fresh berries, a drizzle of honey, and a sprinkle of granola.
- A delicious combination that provides protein, probiotics, and a touch of sweetness.

### 3. Hummus and Veggie Sticks:
- Dip baby carrots, cucumber slices, and bell pepper strips into a portion of hummus.
- A satisfying and nutritious snack rich in fiber and essential nutrients.

### 4. Apple Slices with Nut Butter:
- Slice up an apple and pair it with your favorite nut butter (almond, peanut, or cashew).

- The combination of crisp apple and creamy nut butter offers a delightful mix of textures and flavors.

### 5. Rice Cake Delight:
- Top rice cakes with mashed avocado, cherry tomatoes, and a sprinkle of sea salt.
- A light and cruny snack that provides healthy fats and a burst of freshness.

### 6. Trail Mix Bliss:
- Combine your favorite nuts, dried fruits, and a touch of dark chocolate.
- A portable and satisfying snack that offers a mix of textures and flavors.

### 7. Smoothie Bowl:
- Blend your favorite fruits with yogurt or milk and pour into a bowl.
- Top with granola, chia seeds, and sliced bananas for a refreshing and nutritious snack.

### 8. Cottage Cheese Delight:
- Mix cottage cheese with pineapple chunks or sliced peaches.
- A protein-rich snack that balances creaminess with a hint of sweetness.

### 9. Energy Bites:

- Prepare no-bake energy bites using ingredients like oats, nut butter, honey, and dark chocolate chips.
- A convenient and energizing snack for a quick pick-me-up.

### 10. *Veggie Chips with Guacamole:*
- Make your veggie chips using sweet potatoes, beets, or kale.
- Pair with a side of homemade guacamole for a tasty and nutrient-packed treat.

### 11. *Seaweed Snacking:*
- Enjoy roasted seaweed snacks for a unique combination of umami flavor and crispiness.
- A low-calorie option rich in minerals and vitamins.

### 12. *Dark Chocolate Dipped Strawberries:*
- Dip fresh strawberries in melted dark chocolate.
- A sweet and indulgent treat that satisfies your sweet tooth with antioxidants.

## *Lazy Yogi Snacking Tips:*

### 1. Portion Control:
Be mindful of portion sizes to maintain a healthy balance.

### 2. Hydration:
Stay hydrated by sipping water throughout the day.

### 3. Listen to Your Body:
Pay attention to hunger and fullness cues, allowing your body's needs to guide your snacking.

### 4. Preparation is Key:
Pre-portion snacks or prepare them in advance for easy access.

Snacking as a lazy yogi is all about simplicity, nourishment, and enjoyment. These snack ideas provide a delightful combination of flavors and nutrients to support your well-being on your laid-back yoga journey.

# Hydration for Optimal Performance

In the world of lazy yoga, as in any physical activity, staying well-hydrated is key to supporting optimal performance and overall well-being. In this section, we'll explore the importance of hydration, how it impacts your lazy yoga practice, and practical tips to ensure you stay adequately hydrated.

## 1. The Role of Hydration in Lazy Yoga:

### Maintaining Fluid Balance:
- Hydration is crucial for maintaining the balance of fluids in your body.
- Proper fluid balance supports overall bodily functions, from digestion to temperature regulation.

## 2. Water as Your Lazy Yoga Ally:

### Hydration and Flexibility:
- Well-hydrated muscles and joints are more flexible, contributing to improved ease of movement during lazy yoga.
- Water is essential for lubricating joints, reducing stiffness, and enhancing flexibility.

## 3. Improved Focus and Energy:

### Hydrated Mind, Hydrated Body:

- Dehydration can lead to fatigue, headaches, and a decrease in cognitive function.
- Staying hydrated helps maintain mental clarity, focus, and sustained energy levels.

### 4. Signs of Dehydration to Watch For:

**Listen to Your Body:**
- A dry mouth, dark urine, dizziness, or lethargy can indicate dehydration.
- Pay attention to these signs and address them promptly by rehydrating.

### 5. How Much Water Do You Need?

**Tailor Your Hydration:**
- Individual hydration needs vary based on factors like age, weight, climate, and activity level.
- A general guideline is to aim for about 8 glasses (64 ounces) of water per day, adjusting based on your unique circumstances.

### 6. Timing Your Hydration:

**Pre-Hydration for Lazy Yoga:**
- Drink water before your lazy yoga session to ensure your body starts well-hydrated.
- This helps support flexibility and prevent fatigue during your practice.

**Hydration Throughout the Day:**
- Sip water consistently throughout the day, maintaining a steady level of hydration.
- Waiting until you're thirsty is a reactive approach; aim for proactive hydration.

## 7. Electrolytes and Lazy Yoga:

**Balancing Minerals:**
- Lazy yoga, though gentle, can lead to sweating, particularly in warm environments.
- Replenish electrolytes with options like coconut water or a balanced sports drink, especially if your practice involves light sweating.

## 8. Hydration as a Lifestyle:

**Beyond the Mat:**
- Embrace hydration as a lifestyle, extending beyond your lazy yoga practice.
- Make it a habit to carry a water bottle and take regular sips throughout the day.

## 9. Infusing Flavor into Hydration:

**Herbal Infusions:**
- Add natural flavors to your water with herbal infusions like mint, cucumber, or citrus.
- Experiment with combinations to make hydration enjoyable.

## *10. Celebrating the Benefits of Hydration:*

**Acknowledge Your Well-Hydrated Self:**
- Celebrate the positive impact of hydration on your lazy yoga practice and overall health.
- Recognize the connection between staying hydrated and experiencing the full benefits of your laid-back yoga routine.

### *Lazy Yogi Hydration Success:*
Meet Alex, a dedicated couch potato yogi who prioritized hydration. By incorporating mindful water intake into daily routines, Alex experienced increased flexibility, improved focus during lazy yoga, and enhanced overall well-being.

### *Breaking it Down:*
Hydration is the unsung hero of your lazy yoga journey, supporting flexibility, focus, and energy levels. As we continue on this path, remember that a well-hydrated body is a resilient and energized body. Get ready to raise a metaphorical water bottle to the power of hydration in optimizing your lazy yoga performance and well-being.

# Chapter 8

# Yoga Pro Tips for the Dedicated Couch Potato

## Advanced Lazy Yoga Poses

Congratulations on reaching the advanced stage of your lazy yoga journey! In this chapter, we'll explore pro tips and advanced lazy yoga poses that will challenge your body and mind, taking your practice to new heights while maintaining the laid-back essence that defines the couch potato yogi lifestyle.

### *1. Mindful Progression:*

**Building on Foundations:**
- Advanced lazy yoga poses often build upon the foundations of basic poses.
- Mindfully progress, ensuring you have a strong understanding of the fundamentals before attempting more challenging postures.

### *2. Core Strength for Lazy Yogis:*

**Plank Variations:**

- Explore different plank variations to strengthen your core.
- Side plank, forearm plank, and high plank with leg lifts are excellent options to target core muscles.

### *3. Inversion Exploration:*

**Supported Headstand (Sirsasana):**
- Use a wall for support as you gradually explore the supported headstand.
- This inversion provides a new perspective and enhances upper body strength.

### *4. Balance Challenge:*

**Tree Pose Variation:**
- Elevate the challenge of the tree pose by closing your eyes or extending your arms overhead.
- This variation enhances balance and concentration.

### *5. Hip Opener Intensity:*

**Pigeon Pose (Eka Pada Rajakapotasana):**
- Deepen the hip-opening experience with variations such as king pigeon or mermaid pose.
- These poses require flexibility and mindful breathing to release tension in the hips.

## 6. Advanced Twists:

### Revolved Triangle Pose (Parivrtta Trikonasana):
- Explore advanced twists like the revolved triangle to enhance spinal flexibility.
- Engage your core and twist from the torso, deepening the stretch.

## 7. Arm Balance Play:

### Crow Pose (Bakasana):
- Progress to arm balances like the crow pose, focusing on engaging your core and finding balance in your hands.
- Start with short holds and gradually extend the duration as you gain strength.

## 8. Flexibility Challenges:

### King Pigeon Pose (Raja Kapotasana):
- Deepen your backbend practice with the king pigeon pose.
- Focus on hip flexibility and heart opening in this advanced lazy yoga posture.

## 9. Relaxing into Advanced Restorative Poses:

### Supported Fish Pose (Matsyasana):
- Utilize props to enhance the restorative aspect of the fish pose.

- Support the back and neck while allowing the heart to open for a deeply relaxing experience.

## 10. Consistency and Patience:

### Everyday Progress:
- Consistency is key when exploring advanced poses.
- Celebrate the progress you make each day, even if it's just a subtle improvement in your flexibility or balance.

## 11. Pro Tip - Mindful Breathing:

### Breath Awareness in Advanced Poses:
- Maintain a steady and mindful breath in advanced poses.
- Deep, intentional breathing enhances focus, relaxes the nervous system, and aids in maintaining balance.

## 12. Yoga Pro Success Story:
Meet Jamie, a dedicated couch potato yogi who embraced advanced lazy yoga poses with patience and consistency. Through mindful progression and a commitment to daily practice, Jamie achieved a new level of strength, flexibility, and overall well-being.

### Breaking it Down:
Advanced lazy yoga poses bring a new dimension to your practice, challenging both body and mind. As we move

forward, remember that the journey is as important as the destination. Embrace the advanced poses with a sense of curiosity, patience, and a commitment to the mindful essence of lazy yoga. Get ready to elevate your practice to pro levels, celebrating the achievements of your dedicated couch potato yoga journey.

# Joining Lazy Yoga Classes or Communities

Embarking on the journey of lazy yoga is an exciting venture, and joining classes or communities can add a social and motivational aspect to your practice. In this chapter, we'll explore the benefits of participating in lazy yoga classes or communities, offering insights into how group dynamics can enhance your experience as a dedicated couch potato yogi.

## 1. Community Support:

### A Shared Journey:
- Joining a lazy yoga class or community connects you with like-minded individuals on a similar journey.
- Shared experiences, challenges, and successes create a supportive environment.

## 2. Motivation and Accountability:

### Group Momentum:
- The collective energy of a class or community can motivate you to stay consistent with your lazy yoga practice.
- Knowing that others share your commitment adds a layer of accountability.

### *3. Guided Instruction:*

**Expert Guidance:**
- Lazy yoga classes led by experienced instructors provide expert guidance on poses, alignment, and breathing techniques.
- Personalized feedback ensures you practice safely and effectively.

### *4. Variety in Practice:*

**Diverse Class Offerings:**
- Classes often incorporate a variety of lazy yoga styles, poses, and sequences.
- This diversity prevents monotony, keeping your practice engaging and dynamic.

### *5. Social Connection:*

**Meet Like-minded Individuals:**
- Lazy yoga classes are an opportunity to meet people who share your interest in a laid-back approach to wellness.
- Building connections with fellow couch potato yogis adds a social dimension to your practice.

### *6. Online and In-Person Options:*

**Flexibility in Access:**

- Choose between in-person classes or online platforms based on your preferences and schedule.
- Online classes offer the convenience of practicing from the comfort of your home.

## 7. Community Events:

### Workshops and Gatherings:
- Many lazy yoga communities organize workshops, events, and gatherings.
- These occasions provide opportunities to deepen your practice, learn new techniques, and connect with the community.

## 8. Progress Tracking:

### Celebrate Milestones:
- In a class or community setting, you can track your progress alongside others.
- Celebrating milestones, whether they are improved flexibility or mastering a challenging pose, becomes a collective achievement.

## 9. Supportive Atmosphere:

### Inclusive Environment:
- Lazy yoga communities often foster inclusivity, welcoming individuals of all levels and backgrounds.

- The supportive atmosphere encourages everyone to explore their practice at their own pace.

## *10. Personal Growth:*

### Beyond the Mat:
- Engaging with a lazy yoga class or community can extend beyond the physical practice.
- Shared insights, mindfulness practices, and wellness discussions contribute to your overall personal growth.

## *11. Testimonials and Success Stories:*

### Inspiration from Peers:
- Hearing the stories and successes of fellow lazy yogis can inspire and motivate you.
- Testimonials within the community create a positive and encouraging atmosphere.

## *12. Community Connection Success:*
Meet Taylor, who initially practiced lazy yoga alone. Joining a community not only provided guidance but also introduced Taylor to a supportive network, resulting in enhanced motivation and a more enriched yoga journey.

### *Breaking it Down:*
Joining lazy yoga classes or communities adds a dynamic and enriching layer to your practice. As we move forward, consider exploring these communal

spaces to elevate your experience, share in the collective energy, and celebrate the joys of being part of a couch potato yogi community. Get ready to connect, grow, and thrive on your lazy yoga journey.

# Taking Lazy Yoga Outdoors

Venturing into the great outdoors can breathe new life into your lazy yoga practice, allowing you to connect with nature while embracing the laid-back essence of your journey. In this chapter, we'll explore the benefits of taking lazy yoga outdoors and provide insights on how to infuse the natural world into your practice.

### 1. Nature's Serene Studio:

**Open-Air Tranquility:**
- Practicing lazy yoga outdoors offers a serene and open-air studio.
- The natural surroundings create a calming backdrop for your practice.

### 2. Connection with Nature:

**Earthing Experience:**
- Feeling the earth beneath you enhances the grounding aspect of lazy yoga.
- Direct contact with nature fosters a sense of connection and mindfulness.

### 3. Sunshine and Vitamin D:

**Sun Salutations in Nature:**
- The sun's rays can elevate your energy during lazy yoga.

- Incorporate sun salutations to embrace the warmth and soak in the natural vitamin D.

## *4. Breath of Fresh Air:*

## Oxygenate Your Practice:
- Breathing in fresh outdoor air revitalizes your body and mind.
- Deep, mindful breaths become even more invigorating amidst nature.

## *5. Scenic Inspiration:*

## Visual Delight:
- Surrounding yourself with natural beauty provides visual inspiration.
- Let the scenery enhance your lazy yoga experience, whether it's a park, beach, or forest.

## *6. Gentle Soundscape:*

## Natural Melodies:
- The gentle sounds of birds, rustling leaves, or flowing water create a natural soundscape.
- Allow these soothing sounds to accompany your lazy yoga practice.

## *7. Mindful Grounding Practices:*

## Barefoot Connection:

- If safe and appropriate, practice lazy yoga with bare feet on natural surfaces.
- This tactile experience enhances the grounding and mindfulness aspects of your practice.

## *8. Lazy Yoga Picnic:*

### Combine Relaxation and Nourishment:
- Pack a light picnic and enjoy a post-lazy yoga relaxation amidst nature.
- Connect with the earth, savoring both your practice and a nourishing meal.

## *9. Outdoor Props:*

### Natural Props:
- Utilize natural elements like rocks or logs as props during your lazy yoga practice.
- These additions enhance balance and stability while harmonizing with the outdoor environment.

## *10. Weather-Adaptable Practice:*

### Embrace Seasonal Changes:
- Adjust your lazy yoga practice based on the weather.
- Practice under the warmth of the sun in summer or embrace the crisp air during autumn.

## *11. Group Outdoor Sessions:*

### Community Connection in Nature:
- Organize or join group lazy yoga sessions in outdoor spaces.
- Shared practices in nature foster a sense of community and shared energy.

### *Outdoor Yoga Success Story:*
Meet Alex, a couch potato yogi who discovered the joy of taking lazy yoga outdoors. By practicing in local parks and embracing the changing seasons, Alex found renewed inspiration and a deeper connection to both yoga and nature.

### *Breaking it Down:*
Taking lazy yoga outdoors introduces a harmonious blend of natural elements into your practice, fostering a deeper connection with both your body and the world around you. As we move forward, consider stepping outside to infuse your practice with the beauty and tranquility of nature. Get ready to unroll your mat amidst the great outdoors, embracing the true spirit of lazy yoga in the open air.

# Conclusion

As we conclude this guide, "From Couch Potato to Yoga Pro: The Lazy Person's Step-by-Step Guide to Yoga, Improve Your Health, Fitness, and Well-being," we reflect on the transformative journey you've undertaken as a dedicated couch potato yogi. Throughout these chapters, we've explored the gentle yet powerful world of lazy yoga, discovering how this laid-back approach can bring balance, flexibility, and mindfulness into your life.

From understanding the fundamentals of yoga for lazy beginners to exploring advanced poses, joining communities, and taking your practice outdoors, you've navigated a path that aligns with your unique pace and lifestyle. The lazy yoga journey is not about pushing yourself to extremes but rather about finding harmony and well-being in each intentional, mindful movement.

In the embrace of lazy yoga, you've built strength, enhanced flexibility, and cultivated a sense of inner peace. The community support, expert guidance, and the beauty of nature have enriched your practice, making it a holistic and fulfilling experience. Whether you're a seasoned yogi or just starting your journey, the lazy approach has shown you that wellness is attainable through small, consistent efforts.

As you continue your lazy yoga journey beyond these pages, remember that the essence of this practice lies not in perfection but in the joy of movement, the connection with your breath, and the celebration of your unique progress. The title, "From Couch Potato to Yoga Pro," symbolizes the evolution you've undergone, a testament to the transformative power of lazy yoga in enhancing your health, fitness, and overall well-being.

May your mat always be a sanctuary, a space where you can unroll the wisdom gained from each chapter, breathe in the tranquility of lazy yoga, and carry the essence of this practice into your daily life. Your journey has just begun, and each lazy yoga session is an opportunity to evolve, grow, and celebrate the beautiful and harmonious path you've chosen.

Here's to your continued journey from the couch to the mat, and from the mat to a life filled with well-being, serenity, and the joy of being a proud couch potato yogi. Namaste.